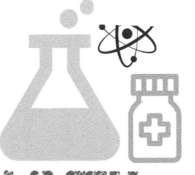

PHARMYTHOLOGY

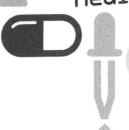

A Pharmacist's Guide to Demystifying Medicine

Zahraa Alalag
Pharm.D, BCMTMS

To Adel and Tamather

Pharmythology: A Pharmacist's Guide to Demystifying Medicine

Published 2023

First Edition

Copyright 2023 Zahraa Alalag

Cover, interior design and illustrations by Simon Thompson.

Contents

Section I
FUNDAMENTAL MYTHS

Section II
MEDICATIONS

Section III
PHARMACY PRACTICE

Prologue

The last 100 years or so have brought a plethora of medical breakthroughs—from milestones in drug regulations, to drug discoveries, and the birth of personalized medicine. But that inevitably created confusion in the way in which health information is communicated.

Reliable and relatable

What motivated me to write this book was witnessing dullness and confusion surrounding medicine. I have wondered if it is possible to communicate information that is reliable and relatable at the same time.

The book is intended to investigate commonly asked questions about medications. Drawing from scientific background, applicable scenarios, and historical tales, it conveys a wide range of intriguing ideas using simple language and an exploratory method.

There are eight chapters, each addressing a central question. The goal is not to discredit an older belief system in lieu of a newer discovery. Instead, the book explores differing schools of thought on various topics, starting from perceptions of how medicine works all the way to assumptions about the healthcare system which are taken for granted. Some answers may gradually reveal themselves as the information slowly builds up, but the takeaway to any question is completely yours to decide.

Suspending judgment

The book has an unassuming nature for a couple of reasons. First, capturing reality from different angles and viewpoints is an enriching experience. There is something to be learned from different schools of thought, be it pharmacogenomics (an emerging practice in modern medicine) or naturopathic medicine (the use of natural remedies).

Today's beliefs are tomorrow's myths

Another reason is to keep an open mind about what we generally accept to be true. This book curiously treats everything we know as a potential myth. Mythology and folk science often get a bad rap (sometimes, for legitimate reasons). But even in the context of evidence-based medicine, perceptions change over time. I see patients who describe bizarre medical practices that occurred only a few decades ago. Someday, our great-grandchildren will look at our current medical practices and wonder: What were they thinking?

Myths: mischievous or misconceived?

When you hear a statement that you know to be false, you may wonder why the misinformation is still going around. But before jumping to debunk and get rid of it, what if it serves as a lens through which to explore the perspectives, fears and tales of others?

Suppose a large group of people believes a certain myth. Perhaps they do so because it has truly worked for them. Or maybe it was once a beneficial belief to a certain group that marked its territory on our current belief system without our realization. For instance, resistance and mistrust of revolutionary tests or treatments are recurring themes in medicine. Today, they can promote fear and can be used to persuade cancer patients to ditch chemotherapy in favor of holistic medicine. But, perhaps staying away from a new treatment or formulation developed by a chemist was a wise thing to do before clinical trials became a thing and FDA regulations were enforced. (More on that in chapter 5)

Is there more to medicine than you know?

This book brushes the surface of many mind-boggling concepts.

Can a drug, for example, unlock your ability to learn a rare musical skill? Or affect your capacity to feel empathy?

Can a pill lower your cholesterol more drastically simply because you expect it to?

What else can you manifest with the 'placebo effect'?

Would you rather take a pill that isn't approved by the FDA but has been safely used for decades, or spend thousands of dollars on the same drug if it were formally evaluated by the FDA?

What else can you derive from pharmaceutical controversies, tragic or lucky coincidences, and honest medical mistakes?

Acknowledgments

I would like to recognize a special group of individuals who have been incredibly supportive of my entire journey from the start all the way through to publication of this book.

I want to thank Simon Thompson, for his creative graphic designs, and David Bamford, for his tremendous encouragement and help throughout the editing process. As a first-time author, I simply couldn't have done this without their support. A special thanks to editor David Haviland, whose talent in this genre is evident in his mind-boggling books. I am grateful for his dedication and help every step of the way.

Thank you to one of my former professors and best mentors, Dr. Goar Alvarez, for all your support. Thanks to my family, especially Aunt Alia, Nafeela, Asia, Khamal, Khuloud, Fadia, Alaa, Hala and Uncle Alaa, Talal, Zaid, and Hameed, whose quality books have inspired me to write ever since I was a child. To everyone who had been a great part of my life: Hinda, Badia, Salaam, Samer, Muhannad, Asmaa, Musaab, Saif, Fatima, Yahya, Haya, Amir, Zainab, Haitham, Ahmad, Mohammad, Mariam, Aseel, Mishmish, Yasa, Olla, Reem, Rania, Rand, Leo, Yasmeen, Malaak, Majito, Sindus, Vannie, Hugo, Soud, Sonia, Nuha, Juju, Fufu and Johnson. Thank you for all the fun times we share and for always helping me find my voice. You all hold a special place in my heart. And lastly, thanks to the talented and beautiful little Bana and Jumana. I love you.

Lastly, Mom and Dad, I have no words to express my gratitude for your endless support and for standing behind every decision I make. Mom, you are the most reassuring person in this world. I don't know how you handle all the craziness that I throw your way. You're my rock. Dad, I still owe my curiosity and love for mystery-solving to all those stories you had told me when I was a small kid. My inner 'private detective' is always there. I love you both. This book is for you.

About the author

Zahraa Alalag is a board-certified MTM specialist. She obtained her doctorate degree in pharmacy (Pharm.D) from Nova Southeastern University in South Florida, USA. She works closely with patients with chronic health conditions to prevent medication errors and simplify complex medication regimens.

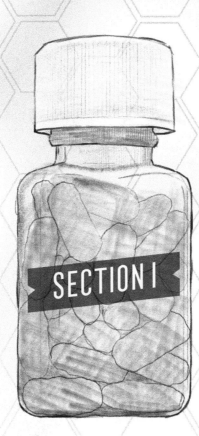

SECTION I

Fundamental Myths

Chapter 1:
How much do you know about your medicine?

If you are reading this book, you probably know a great deal about what goes into your body. Predictability and precision are what we all strive for in modern science, be it in pharmaceuticals, cosmetics, or nutrition. We educate ourselves every day with the hope of achieving a sense of certainty about what we consume. The question of whether we're in for a surprise raises concerns in most of us—patients, clinicians, and scientists alike.

Through my practice, I have come to be familiar with the assumption that clinicians must know everything about their fields. I sometimes get asked questions that, frankly, I do not have answers for yet. As a drug expert, I am certainly alert to the major long-term side effects, tolerability, dependence, dosing regimens, and interactions of medicinal drugs. Yet I do not know everything there is to know about medications.

The following passage will illustrate the level of uncertainty that is sometimes faced even by experts. The rest of the chapter presents a wider selection of drug oddities and unexpected consequences.

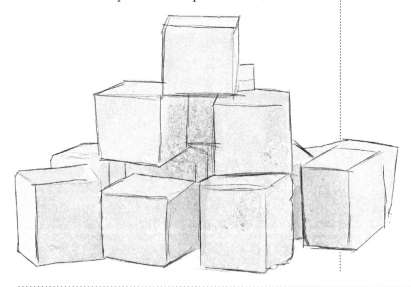

The sweet taste of chemistry

One evening in Baltimore, in February 1878, Constantin Fahlberg had just gotten home from a long day at his lab. He was a knowledgeable chemist who worked on coal tar derivatives at Johns Hopkins University. After working for endless hours, he was so fatigued that he immediately rushed for comfort food. After taking a few bites of bread, he was startled by how sweet it tasted. He looked at his hands and observed fine particles of white powder. Instead of washing his hands, this sparked curiosity in the chemist's mind. He started tracking the powder back and tasting everything he had laid his hands on. [1]

Legend has it that this is how a popular sugar substitute was discovered. Of course, nobody wants a spoonful of anhydroorthosulphaminebenzoic in their coffee, so it is now referred to as saccharin.

As bizarre as it may seem, many commonly used drugs were discovered by accident. The process of drug discovery isn't always a straightforward or simple one. Sometimes, a drug is observed to be useful, but its mechanism of action remains unknown. Other times, a known drug leads to unpredictable outcomes. The former scenario often leads to unexpected discoveries about the drug, the disease state, or human physiology all together.

Just like in other science fields, knowledge in pharmacology is not written on stone, as it continues to change and evolve. It is a product of years of trial and error, accidental discoveries, drug recalls, educated guesses and erroneous assumptions.

> ## "There is another element which some call luck and others call serendipity, or discovery through the 'happy accident.' I would urge you never to ignore the unusual."
>
> — John Vane[2]

"It is not me; it is my pill."

Most of us are not intrepid explorers like Fahlberg. Nevertheless, there is a good chance of discovering something interesting about any medicine we consume.

For instance, suppose that you started a medication to treat a hand tremor, only to turn into a compulsive shopper or a gambling addict. This may seem laughable at first. But a quick google search can reveal several lawsuits filed against manufacturers of dopamine agonists, a class of anti-parkinsonism drugs. One of the side effects of dopamine agonists is reduced impulse control.

Perhaps, it is not realistic to blame dopamine agonists for all the crimes, gambling, and other addiction issues that exist today. But when you consider the pharmacology, their influence on impulsive control will no longer be a mystery. (More on dopaminergic effects is covered in chapter 8).

> Some pharmaceutical companies have had to pay settlements to compensate the torn families of the individuals who had obsessively gambled their savings away as a result of taking anti-parkinsonism drugs.[3]

Take another example:

Can a popular pain medicine sold over the counter make people less empathic? Imagine caring less for a friend only because you took a painkiller that contained acetaminophen. A research paper titled "A Social Analgesic? Acetaminophen (Paracetamol) Reduces Positive Empathy" published by a team of pain researchers explored this phenomenon.[4] Pain isn't only physical. Reacting to your own emotions, as well as the emotions of others, may be affected by the painkiller, acetaminophen. But there are other surprising effects of taking this drug. Some studies have demonstrated that acetaminophen can induce risky behaviors. This led scientists to believe that pain is an integral part of decision-making as well.[5]

Because acetaminophen reduces pain by acting on the central nervous system (CNS), experiencing mild personality changes is not a surprising side effect. But given how this medicine is easily accessible as an over-the-counter product and how it is commonly used, the consequences of taking it (e.g., partaking in risky behaviors, or lacking empathy, an essential ingredient for human connection) are more troubling than the logic.

But not all side effects are harmful. An intriguing example is a recent study showing a seizure medication can enhance one's ability to acquire a musical talent.[6]

When one door closes, you can reopen the closed door

Absolute pitch is the ability to accurately identify or produce musical notes by ear.[7] Someone with absolute pitch will listen to music and correctly identify the notes that are played. Absolute pitch is so rare that we traditionally attribute it to musical prodigies, like Mozart. It is truly a gift that every aspiring musician wishes to have.

The odds of obtaining absolute pitch are very low: 1 out of 10,000 people, to be exact.

There are several compelling theories on acquiring the absolute pitch.

According to the most popular theory, there is a fixed "critical window" to develop absolute pitch, which closes before the age of 4-6 years.[8]

Much like our bones' ability to grow when we are kids, our young brains have an elasticity—to change, or to acquire talents. This theory implies that we are no longer capable of developing absolute pitch once that window closes.

However, some experts have recently come to reject the idea of a "fixed window" of opportunities, based on evidence of humans' ability to acquire talents at an older age. This is attributed to the brain's ability for rewiring, which seems possible later in life.

The phenomenon of brain rewiring continues to drive debate. But we might be looking at a valid proof for it right in the following instance:

In 2013, a team of researchers hit the headlines with a research paper titled "Valproate reopens critical-period learning of absolute pitch". They demonstrated that when adult volunteers (who did not have absolute pitch) were given valproate (as opposed to placebo), they were able to demonstrate this ability, despite not having any musical training prior to the study.

It is exciting to see that adults can learn absolute pitch, a phenomenon that was deemed impossible until the paper came out.

But the implications for this are rather more profound — re-opening windows for us to obtain unattainable skills and challenge assumptions we have long accepted about our limitations.

Valproic acid is a drug that is used to treat seizure and mood disorders. It has many reported side effects, but acquiring musical skills was not an acknowledged effect until the publication of this paper.

As you can see, unforeseen consequences are common. So much so that an entire innovative field in pharmacology, 'drug repurposing,' exists for the sole purpose of finding uses for drugs beyond their original purposes.

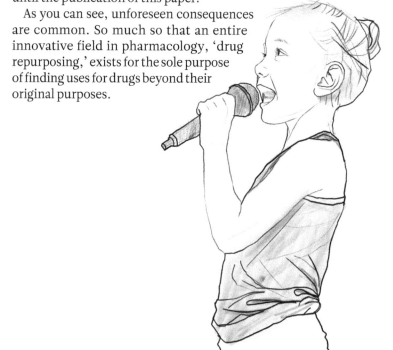

One person's side effect is another's treatment

Since drugs can have various effects, manufacturers also market them for various uses, adding more nuance to the picture.

Nonetheless, they can be quite artful.

Take antihistamines, a class of medicine used to fight allergies. They exert their actions by blocking the effect of histamine, a natural substance released in response to allergens.

Patients are advised to refrain from driving after taking antihistamines, because antihistamines can penetrate the brain and cause side effects (sedation, drowsiness, and cognitive impairment) and increase the risks for falls and driving accidents. In response to these concerns, pharmaceutical companies developed newer generations of antihistamines with diminished ability to penetrate the brain. This is the idea behind "non-drowsy" allergy pills.

Yet, despite newer generations, good old diphenhydramine, a first-generation antihistamine, remains the traditional ingredient used in cold medicines.

Why is that that?

Adding diphenhydramine in PM formulations helps a patient recover from a cold by making them fall asleep.

Drowsiness is a negative side effect in allergy medicine, but it is a desired outcome when used in cold medicine. One substance is not necessarily good or bad until you put it in the context of its intended patient group and therapeutic goal.

Post meridiem (PM) is the Latin term for "after midday". PM formulations like Advil PM or Tylenol PM are intended to be used in the evening or at bedtime.

Chapter 2

Does your genetic makeup influence your response to medicine?

Is your genetic blueprint currently influencing your drug response as you are reading this book?

Everyone wants to feel certain about their medications. It is certainly not an area in which people welcome the idea of being uncertain or adventurous.

Or is it?

Imagine a technology that could determine which drugs you should be taking to prevent catastrophes twenty years down the road, like heart disease, strokes, or cancers. Or what if, upon receiving a new diagnosis at your doctor's office, your genetic information could instantly generate a list of medications you would be likely to respond well to, and a list of medications you should avoid. It's like a scene taken straight from the movie Gattaca.

In a nutshell, Gattaca revolves around a future in which extreme genetic enhancement is considered mainstream. The lead character, constantly reminded of his imperfect genetic make-up, goes to extreme measures to live the life he desires by hijacking someone else's DNA. This fictional movie shows a glimpse of a future that seems improbable and intriguing.

This chapter will explore the overlap between genetics and pharmacology. It will also present the challenges and ethical dilemmas surrounding medical genetics.

The field of genetics has revolutionized not only how we practice medicine, but also the way we understand the world. Yet, given the relatively recent discovery of DNA, the field is relatively young and hence it navigates through new concepts. No one knows with absolute certainty why the largest chunk of our DNA even exists.

> 99% of our noncoding DNA, that had been long dismissed and referred to as 'junk DNA', was discovered to have an important role in cell function and gene activity. Junk DNA may in fact be an integral part of the genome—perhaps in ways that we still do not fully understand.

With that in mind, it is safe to say that the field's most promising prospects are likely still untapped.

Yet, the incorporation of genomic data into medical practice is happening as we speak. Just not to the extent of sci-fi movies... not yet anyway.

Consider the following case:

A woman experienced severe pain after giving birth. She was given a painkiller that contained codeine. She was taking the medicine while breastfeeding the baby. This led to a tragedy, as the drug was subsequently deemed to have caused the baby's death.[9]

> Codeine reduces pain by sedating the central nervous system (CNS). It does that by primarily acting on opioid receptors.
>
> Aside from pain perception, opioids are known for their complexity and diversity of functions that they mediate. High concentration of opioids can cause brain regions responsible for ventilation to ultimately shut down, a condition termed opioid-induced respiratory depression.[10]

Many health professionals tend to steer away from giving opioids to patients that are sensitive to their side effects. Codeine is no exception, even though it was once commonly used even among nursing mothers. This case changed the way that codeine is prescribed in this population. In fact, the drug raised far more controversies and warnings than other opioids, even though it is not as potent as other members of the opioid family.

Many medical and scientific papers started raising concerns about codeine use in nursing mothers, as a small portion of the drug seems to be excreted into the mothers' milk. These concerns led the FDA to issue warnings strongly advising nursing mothers to avoid codeine and its structurally related opioid, tramadol, during breastfeeding.[11, 12]

But there is more to this than the mere association between breastfeeding and the drug.

Codeine is a prodrug of CYP2D6.[13]

A prodrug is an inactive substance that is metabolized by the body to produce the active drug.

In another words, codeine is inactive by itself. Upon ingestion, it gets metabolized by an enzyme called CYP2D6. Subsequently, CYP2D6 turns it into its active form.

CYP2D6 is a member of the cytochrome (CYP450) family. CYP2D6 metabolizes a range of commonly prescribed medications. Some people carry genetic mutations that alter these enzymes—rendering them more or less active than the original ("normal") version.

For most mothers, the risk for adverse events is minimal. But in this case, the mother was found to be an ultra-metabolizer. Ultra-metabolizers are born with a hyperactive variant of the CYP2D6 enzyme, which generates more of codeine's active metabolite. Consequently, ultra-metabolizers will experience more side effects compared to an average person. In this circumstance, an unexpected overdose is a concerning possibility.

These genetic differences carry significant implications. A simple mutation can determine the severity of side effects or whether a drug works in the first place.

Sister morphine

Most people are familiar with morphine and codeine. What many don't realize is that they're twin sisters.

Morphine is the readily active form of codeine after it gets processed by CYP2D6. Only about 10% of codeine is said to be converted to morphine. But this is an average percentage that does not take interindividual genetic differences in drug metabolism into account. In other words, without knowing someone's genetic makeup, prescribing them codeine can feel like a gamble. [14]

The medical community continues raising questions and concerns about genetic mutations and medications. But problems are not always readily recognized or adequately addressed. Consider the reverse of the previous case, for instance, a poor metabolizer, who may not experience any benefit from the medication. This would be more subtle and challenging to diagnose, especially within specialties like pain management or psychopharmacology which deal with many subjective outcomes like pain and mood disorders.

> Every time someone takes codeine, they are essentially taking an undetermined dose of morphine.

Ultimately, we cannot prevent the genetic gamble. It is a part of life. But there's good news: many incidents can be predicted with precision medicine.

Moving away from one pill fits all

Once confined to science fiction, the idea of 'precision medicine' is now a firmly established part of modern pharmaceutical practice.

Here, the term "precision" seems a bit uncanny. Shouldn't every healthcare provider strive to provide treatments in a precise manner?

'Precision medicine' is used interchangeably with 'individualized medicine'. Whichever title appeals to you, the premise here is to have everyone receive the most customized healthcare possible based on their individual differences. The foundation of an individualized care plan looks something like this:

Drug A may work perfectly well for person A.

Drug A does not work so well for person B.

Drug A may present dangers to person C.

Person B and person C may therefore benefit from therapy modification or being put on different drugs in the first place.

This is where pharmacogenomics serves its greatest purpose. Pharmacogenomics is simply the study of how a person's drug response is affected by their genetic makeup. As a field, it translates a patient's genetic information to predictable patterns of drug response.

Indeed, what once started out as an abstract molecular science is now being incorporated into clinical practice in a clinically relevant manner.

Precision Medicine Initiative

In 1990, an international collaborative initiative known as The Human Genome Project was set up to sequence the entire human genome. Initially, the initiative encountered skepticism from biologists and clinicians who were doubtful about its value. Nevertheless, the initiative gained the collaboration of many academics across the globe who aimed to identify as much of human DNA as possible. The project started to map out DNA base pairs (More on DNA base pairs below). It also made this information available to be used as reference for research purposes. By the time the project was completed in 2003, roughly 3.2 billion DNA base pairs had been identified and sequenced.[15]

DNA STRUCTURE

DNA is essentially a set of detailed instructions telling the cells how to work and survive. DNA consists of two linked strands. The backbone of each strand is made of alternating sugar and phosphate groups. Each sugar is attached to one of the four main bases: adenine (A), cytosine (C), guanine (G) or thymine (T).

Each base is paired with another base from the corresponding strand in a specific fashion (adenine is linked to thymine, and cytosine is linked to guanine). In other words, the base pairs (A-T or G-C) are what keep the two strands linked together.

Despite increased interest in genetics research, the United States was still seeing increasing prevalence of obesity and diabetes at that time, and hence was in a great need for preventive and tailored medicine. In 2015, President Obama launched a campaign, the Precision Medicine Initiative, to support the practice of individualized medicine and increase the availability of genetic testing. Throughout the years, genetic testing also became cheaper as DNA sequencing technology also became more efficient.

But many concerns started surfacing around pharmacogenomics. Is individualized medicine practical to apply? Cheaper does not necessarily mean that genetic testing would be affordable for everybody, and there are far greater problems to consider besides cost. For example, will the public accept this as a new practice? Will health practitioners be fully comfortable embracing it? Will health insurance plans support and reimburse institutions for performing these tests? Will clinical guidelines specifically address them? Will there be any other practical implications?

The matter of practicality remains a topic for debate. As a pharmacogenetics enthusiast, I have encountered a wide range of opinions that have ultimately challenged my own take on the subject. I recall an uplifting and reassuring conversation I had with Craig Venter, the founder of Celera Genomics, The Institute for Genomic Research (TIGR). As a synthetic biologist, he believes that the practice of precision medicine (in other words, incorporating molecular medicine into practice) is inevitable. Yet some practitioners I know are still concerned about pharmacogenomic testing as the tests are expensive and often take days and hence can create harmful delays in situations that require urgent treatments.

This isn't to say that clinicians don't believe in the benefits of pharmacogenomics or in the fact that it works. Rather, they are concerned about practical outcomes. Additionally, some are concerned about unforeseen consequences as the field is still relatively new.

Taboos

Despite the controversies, DNA testing is already being integrated in our life. Many people are ordering DNA tests to explore their ancestry and learn about health risks they inherited. Your pharmacist may already be able to order a pharmacogenomics test for you in some circumstances. Of course, this practice may or may not be standardized, depending on where you currently live.

Currently, the most relevant question is whether we (specifically, our healthcare and legal systems) are equipped and ethical enough to handle these breakthroughs.

Imagine that you are asked to do a genetic test, only to later learn that you are being discriminated against. Organizations take many measures to keep DNA information strictly private. But there is no guarantee that data will be protected from leakage, or kept from third parties or law enforcement.

At the very minimum, genetic tests must run in a way that is private and safe.

You might be familiar with the case of "Golden State Killer" which surfaced in the news when the police appeared to find their suspect by accessing the database of GEDmatch, a company that sells DNA test kits. [16]

GEDmatch works in a similar fashion as other companies that people use under the impression that their information stays private. Other companies that target consumers directly (e.g. sell products or testing kits to consumers online) were in fact recently investigated by the Federal Trade Commission for privacy related concerns. [17]

With these concerns in mind, it isn't surprising that genetic testing is unsettling for many. But some might argue that we are assuming a similar risk every time we sign our rights away to do any kind of test or medical procedure.

What makes a genetic test different from a routine blood test as far as privacy risks are concerned? Perhaps the issue is that DNA feels more personal. It can be more incriminating.

Can information extracted from a routine blood test, for instance, ever be used against you?

The possibility of that scenario happening might seem slim. But information such as blood chemistry, nutritional status and hormonal levels are unique in the sense that they can (reliably or unreliably) explain or predict people's behaviors at any given time.

In essence, any medical condition can be brought up

in court. Theoretically, any health-related information, whether it's your hormonal status or even a dip in your blood sugar, can be used to tip a court's decision against you (or in your favor).[18] [19]

So why then do we undoubtedly undergo routine health screenings despite privacy concerns? Because we have faith that our judicial system is competent in its determination of what counts as evidence or grounds for criminal liability.

Some of the implications mentioned in this chapter are more based on slippery slopes rather than solid concerns. But such questions are worth entertaining if they can highlight the idea that any practice has its fair share of unforeseen consequences that people will eventually learn to control as they get familiar with it in the longer run.

Chapter 3
How impactful are drug interactions?

Can you tell if your medications can interact with each another?

It goes without saying that this is a question to investigate with your pharmacist. But a layperson's way to roughly assess your risk for a drug interaction is by counting your medication bottles.

36% of people who are between the age of 62 to 85 years old are reported to be receiving at least 5 prescriptions in the United States.[20] The increased use of medicine is often attributed to a growing elderly population, in addition to increased chronic disease treatments.

However, despite medical advances and increased access to treatments, the number of adverse drug events reported to the FDA doubled between 2006 and 2014.[21] What makes polypharmacy—the use of multiple drugs—particularly problematic is the fact that it increases risks for drug interactions and unforeseen adverse events. 10% of patients in emergency rooms are predicted to encounter a drug interaction each time a new medicine is added.[22]

This chapter provides an overview of various types of drug interactions and explains their mechanisms. Additionally, it uses common clinical scenarios to explore consequences of drug interactions and polypharmacy.

So, what exactly is a drug interaction?

It is any reaction that occurs between the drug and another drug, food, or a disease state.

Additionally, it's important to consider this for a working definition:

Pharmacists suspect that a significant interaction is at play when they observe a change in a drug effect that correlates with an alteration to any variables mentioned above.

The forbidden fruit

Grapefruit juice is a nutritious antioxidant. But it is also known to interact with commonly used medications.

The way in which grapefruit juice can interact with medicine was discovered by accident.[23] In the late 1980s, a team of pharmacologists were trying to evaluate the drug interaction between ethanol and felodipine, a blood pressure medicine. They found greater blood pressure reduction than expected when grapefruit juice was used as a flavor.

Ideally, people with high blood pressure use medications to lower it or keep it under control. However, a steep drop in blood pressure is considered a harmful side effect. An extremely low blood pressure occurs when a high dose of the blood pressure medicine is used, or as a result of a drug interaction that causes the drug level in the body to increase.

The experiment immediately drove focus on grapefruit juice as it was suspected to have caused a change (an increase) in felodipine's level and consequently, its effect. Not surprisingly, that was confirmed in subsequent studies. Since then, the scientific community acknowledges that grapefruit juice can influence medication levels.

Grapefruit juice is now a recognized inhibitor of CYP3A4. CYP3A4 is responsible for eliminating felodipine.

In other words, grapefruit juice can increase felodipine's level by slowing down its elimination. As a result, it can intensify the side effects (too much drop in blood pressure).

Should you worry about grapefruit juice?

Given that CYP3A4 is said to metabolize over 1900 drugs, patients often wonder if they should stop drinking grapefruit juice.[24]

The extent to which grapefruit juice can affect observable clinical outcomes is widely variable. Some studies did not observe significant negative outcomes, whereas other studies noticed increased toxicities of CYP3A4 substrates when grapefruit is combined.

This picture is further complicated by other factors. First, unpredictable responses could occur because people metabolize drugs differently. Second, there is no way to standardize the composition of grapefruit juice because it's natural (not a pharmaceutical product).

Whether you should reduce grapefruit juice intake or avoid it depends on the specific case. The consensus on this varies from monitoring or limiting intake of large quantities of grapefruit juice to prohibiting certain combinations altogether.

The bitter side of macrolides

Imagine receiving an antibiotic for a chest infection, only to develop severe muscle pain shortly after your doctor visit.

You may write off the body ache as a side effect of the cholesterol pill you happen to take, simvastatin. (More on statins' side effects in chapter 7). Or perhaps it could be the result of the infection itself. Or both. But if the new medicine happens to be erythromycin, then it might have also greatly contributed to the problem.

> Erythromycin belongs to macrolides, a family of antibiotics commonly used for lung infections. Erythromycin is also a strong CYP3A4 inhibitor.[25]

As an inhibitor, it intensifies toxicities of simvastatin, which happens to be metabolized by CYP3A4.[26]

Although rare, this combination may even lead to rhabdomyolysis, muscle damage so severe that one's muscles break down and release their inner contents into the bloodstream. This process can overtax the kidneys as they try to eliminate the waste, and hence can lead to further injury, and potentially death, if not treated as an emergency. It is a rare incident, but it happens. In fact, this scenario somewhat resembles the real-life case of an 85-year-old man who received erythromycin for pneumonia and ended up in the emergency room with a case of rhabdomyolysis due to the drug interacting with simvastatin.[27]

Ideally, you should always be warned about this possible drug interaction ahead of time.

If you live in the United States, it is a legal requirement that you are at least presented with an opportunity to speak with the pharmacist when you receive a prescription. This is usually included in the paperwork received with a medication or the electronic signature pad that you sign off before paying. Many patients sign this without realizing that they're waiving their right to pharmacist-patient counseling that could be life saving.

Can an antidepressant have an effect on cancer survival?

Suppose a woman takes an antidepressant, bupropion, while receiving tamoxifen for breast cancer treatment.

A common form of breast cancer needs estrogen to proliferate, necessitating a drug like tamoxifen to stop it from growing.

But tamoxifen is inactive. Like codeine, it is a prodrug of CYP2D6.[28] It gets converted to endoxifen, the active substance. Endoxifen then binds to estrogen receptors and inhibits them from fueling cancer growth.

> Tamoxifen is a hormonal therapy that blocks estrogen receptors.

Bupropion, the antidepressant used in this case, happens to inhibit CYP2D6. It can therefore hinder tamoxifen's activation.[29]

What does this mean for this patient? The medication that she is taking to shrink her tumor may not be effective.

Given the prevalent diagnosis of depression in cancer patients, practitioners are often careful to avoid this combination as it may disrupt cancer treatment protocols and affect survival for cancer patients.

But drug interactions are often more complex than they appear. For example, in the case of tamoxifen, some may argue that it is also metabolized by other enzymes. Thus, a CYP2D6 inhibitor is not necessarily going to alter the patient's overall chance of survival. But I have not met a clinician willing to take such a major risk unnecessarily. This is especially true given the availability of other options of antidepressants that can be used without risking this interaction.

A CYP of medicine

It's easy to see why cytochrome P450 enzymes play such an important role in pharmacology. Notice, for example, that if you were to replace the genetic difference that had caused the mother mentioned in the previous chapter to be a CYP hyper-metabolizer with a drug that induces the enzyme, the results would be the same. (at least in principle).

Sometimes people's genetics cause them to metabolize drugs differently, other times the cause can be a medicine they take or a juice they drink. The common denominator, however, is the role of a CYP enzyme.

A CLOSER LOOK AT WHAT HAPPENS DURING DRUG METABOLISM

As drugs go through the liver, they undergo a series of biochemical reactions. This happens with the help of the CYP enzymes, which are predominately present in the liver.

After being processed by the cytochrome enzymes, most drugs get inactivated and subsequently eliminated from the body. (Think of the classic role of the liver as a detoxification organ)

But prodrugs are an exception. They become more active than the parent drug after encountering the enzymes.

You may think of a prodrug's dependence on the CYP enzyme as a form of hindrance (it's as if they need a key switch to be turned on).

But pharmacologists look at it a bit differently. They can now utilize these variances in drug metabolism to improve drug delivery and enhance targeted drug therapies, for instance. To a strategic drug designer, this is the exact step that is going to shield the drug from biochemical destruction or rapid elimination before it reaches its primary target.

Up to this point, the drug interactions I presented are relatively easy to spot (and prevent). What about interactions caused by polypharmacy?

Heartburns and heart attacks

Suppose that you start taking aspirin because your doctor has recommended it to prevent heart attacks. A few weeks later, you begin to experience an upset stomach. A month later, this issue progresses to more than an occasional heartburn. What would you expect to happen?

Not everyone survives a cardiovascular event. And the ones who survive face challenges to reduce heart damage and prevent recurrences. Taking a blood thinner like aspirin to prevent a vascular event before it happens seems like a brilliant investment. Aspirin is a blood thinner that is available in low doses (81 mg) for anyone to purchase over the counter.

But aspirin is a major gastric irritant. In fact, when someone says aspirin "pokes a hole" in their stomach, they probably experience that in the literal sense. People often quit taking aspirin because it has caused them to have stomach ulcers.

Aspirin blocks the synthesis of two cyclooxygenase enzymes (COX-1 and COX-2). The cyclooxygenase enzymes produce biologically active substances, namely prostaglandins and thromboxanes.

Prostaglandins and thromboxanes are important for survival as well as for regular, day-to-day functions. For instance, they help form blood clots and are involved in inflammation. By blocking their production, aspirin works as a blood thinner and a fever reducer.[30]

Aspirin's bothersome effects stem from the fact that it disrupts the stomach's natural lining which is formed by prostaglandins. When taking aspirin, the stomach is left with less protective 'cushion' against irritation or ulcers.

So, the question becomes: How much discomfort would you be willing to tolerate to continue taking aspirin?

On a larger scale, this dilemma constantly urges health associations to draw the line at which the benefit of preventing a heart attack would outweigh the risk of a life threating ulcer.[31] Aspirin recommendations have been constantly refined to target appropriate patient population. In other words, recommending aspirin is balanced act that considers everyone's age and health status.

But the next question is, how do you keep people motivated to take it?

This is where the usefulness of acid suppressants comes into the picture. Agents like histamine H2-receptor antagonists (H2-blockers) or proton pump inhibitors (PPIs) can shield the stomach from irritation and ulceration caused by aspirin.

In this case, the effect of one drug reduces (or cancels out) the effect of another drug. This scenario can be useful if carefully tailored and monitored.

But what would happen if several years pass by and you continue taking aspirin with the acid reducer? Maybe nothing happens. Or maybe you wake up one day to the realization that you are taking too many medications to compensate for the consequences of taking aspirin.

Polyphony of problems: Polypharmacy

Suppose that you take aspirin plus a proton pump inhibitor (PPI) for years. You might brush it off and think, 'What can go wrong?'

Osteoporosis, pneumonia, and muscle cramps are just part of a list of effects associated with prolonged use of proton pump inhibitors (PPIs).[32] [33] We can focus on one side effect for the sake of argument: osteoporosis.

Because PPIs decrease stomach acidity, they can reduce the body's ability to absorb nutrients that rely on the acidic environment of the stomach for proper absorption. One of those happens to be calcium, which is an important mineral for bone health.

This is how chronic PPI use can increase the risk of osteoporosis.

To combat that, suppose that, like many people, you end up on an agent that reduces bone loss, like alendronate.

It would only take a couple of weeks of use to learn that alendronate is a harsh stomach irritant.

Alendronate and aspirin are said to have additive toxicity. This is a type of drug interaction that's observed when the effects of one drug is increased by another drug (often acting in a similar manner or having similar toxicities).

Polypharmacy often starts from an innocent initiative to be healthier but leads to cases that are inevitably difficult to manage because the effects of different drugs (overlapping side effects) can get tangled quickly.

A common concern patients express during MTM appointments is that they feel they are taking too many medications. It can be stressful, financially draining, and difficult to manage. Some people cannot even recall how it all started or why some drugs were given to them in the first place.

These previous examples are presented here to shed some light on the nature of polypharmacy. These cases exist on a continuous spectrum. At one end of the spectrum, you could have a beneficial and simple symbiotic combination. At the other end, you could have an ever-mounting sequence of medications and adverse effects. And for that reason, complex drug regimens are best to evaluate on a case-by-case basis.

"Drugs are of priceless value when needed, but they are at best emergency measures of most temporary utility... The more effective they are in the right place, the more harmful in the wrong one."

— Woods Hutchinson.[34]

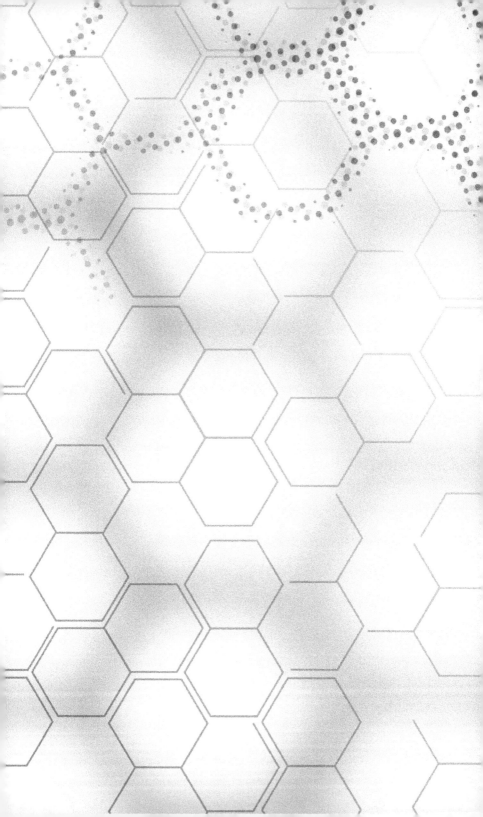

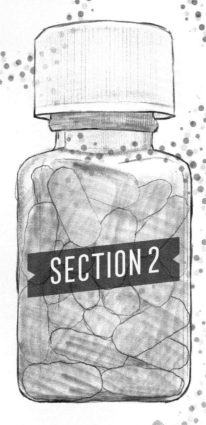

SECTION 2

Medications

Chapter 4
Do natural supplements work? And are they safe?

Have you ever wondered how far some of the genuine ancient remedies have come to be on our pharmacy counters, both geographically and historically?

The use of natural products evokes strong opposing opinions (especially among clinicians) as many doubt their efficacy and safety.

This chapter explores real stories and clinical cases to reveal 'the good, bad and the ugly' sides of natural medicine. It also demonstrates innovative drug design ideas that stemmed from nature.

Despite the controversies, natural medicine is nothing short of a celebration of human curiosity and innovation. Natural remedies have been used for centuries by millions of our ancestors around the globe. The notion of deriving medicine from an animal, classically a snake, is ancient. It is evident in the classic Caduceus sign, which now is used as a symbol of health professions across the globe.

From toxins to life-saving drugs: Delivered by nature

What makes a snake's venom popular today? Look no further for it than in your medicine bottles.

The blood pressure pill we now call captopril was originally extracted from the Brazilian pit viper, Bothrops jararaca.

In fact, if your blood pressure pill ends with "pril", then you have the Brazilian pit viper to thank. Through their venom, these snakes are thought to kill their prey by drastically dropping the blood pressure.

How?

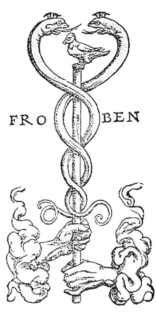

The caduceus trademark with the two intertwining snakes portraited in works of the Swiss medical printer, Johann Frobenius.[35]

This question fascinated John Vane, the pharmacologist who later won the Nobel Prize in Physiology or Medicine in 1982 for his discoveries on prostaglandins (he is the person who discovered how aspirin works to prevent clots). At that time, John Vane worked closely with a Brazilian scientist, Sérgio Ferreira, to understand the chemical properties of the snake's venom.

The team discovered that the ingredient they extracted from the venom caused a drop in blood pressure by inhibiting angiotensin converting enzyme (ACE), an enzyme that controls blood pressure. This is how the popular class of drugs we now call "ACE inhibitors" were developed.[36] ACE also turns out to have a role in heart and kidney health.

It is clear to see how this discovery revolutionized cardiovascular medicine. It also unlocked a new understanding on how blood pressure works in the first place.

But snakes aren't the only natural source of drugs. New diabetes medications, glucagon-like peptide (GLP-1) agonists, come from a lizard's venom.[37]

> ACE inhibitors are a drug class commonly used to lower blood pressure. In addition to that, they are now used to slow down heart remodeling (aging) after heart attacks, and to prevent kidney damage in diabetic patients.

This venom doesn't necessarily kill, but it seems to have a paralyzing (immobilization) effect. When scientists extracted the ingredient, they discovered that it lowers blood sugar. Eventually, the first GLP-1 agonist, exenatide, was developed. Similar GLP-1 agonists were later synthesized based on the same molecule.

Glucagon-like peptide (GLP-1) agonists can also curb appetite. In fact, in 2021, the FDA approved another drug in this family, semaglutide (Wegovy, Novo Nordisk) to be used for weight loss.[38]

Glucagon-like peptide (GLP-1) agonists in weight loss: Beyond cosmetics?

We have many medications to treat diabetes nowadays. But glucagon-like peptide (GLP-1) agonists are a game changer because of their ability to help with weight loss.

Think of how obesity, diabetes and cardiovascular events are all interconnected. Glucagon-like peptide (GLP-1) agonists might be better than insulin therapy, the standard injectable therapy for diabetes.

Why? Weight gain is a commonly reported side effect of insulin injections, which can be particularly counterproductive when they are used by obese patients or by anyone who struggles to lose weight.

ACE inhibitors and glucagon-like peptide (GLP-1) agonists are now commonly prescribed. Prescription medications are strictly evaluated by the FDA. Herbals products, however, are not regulated by the FDA to the same extent as prescription drugs.

The controversial flower

Take St John's wort, a plant-based remedy used for over a century to treat depression. Many doctors in the USA feel uneasy about this supplement. But it is still used to treat various conditions throughout the world to this day. It is most widely used as a mood booster. It is also known to be an anti-inflammatory remedy and a painkiller.

St John's wort was recently found to be more effective than placebo and to have similar effectiveness to standard medicinal treatment of depression in an analysis of 23 randomized trials.[40] Nonetheless, high-quality evidence on this is still lacking.

> St John's wort elevates mood by inhibiting the re-uptake (reabsorption) of the neurotransmitters serotonin, norepinephrine, and dopamine.

So, why is it dismissed by health professionals, if it can be useful in some cases?

The practice of medicine in the west has shifted from many traditions that might still be celebrated elsewhere as western practitioners now favor pharmaceutical products with standardized doses, purity and concentration, rather than naturally-occurring products.

There are various reasons for this.

Firstly, most practitioners are simply not trained to use herbals to a degree that allows them to comfortably have discussions about natural remedies.

St John's wort has various uses and ancient roots. Its Latin name, Hypericum perforatum, hints at the plant's association with magical properties. The term "Hypericum perforatum" is derived from Greek and thought to mean "above apparition" as the plant was used against evil or supernatural forces thousands of years ago.[39]

Secondly, the purity of herbal preparations cannot be standardized or predicted with precision. In fact, without strict oversight from the FDA, some St John's wort products you can buy online might be fake, for all you know.

Lastly, some natural products tend to cause serious drug interactions and adverse events. This is the main reason why St John's wort products—or other herbals—are concerning for many pharmacists.

For instance, take the case of a man who found a matching donor after years waiting for a liver transplant. Fourteen months after the transplant, he was hospitalized for a severe case of organ rejection.

What led to that event?

It was discovered that he started using St John's wort a few weeks prior to the incident.[41]

Consider the details of this case: To prevent organ rejection, he was taking cyclosporin, an immunosuppressant.

When an organ is transplanted, it registers as a foreign substance in the body of transplant recipient. Immunosuppressants, like cyclosporin, are vital to the survival of transplant recipients as they prevent the immune system from attacking the new organ, which can lead to organ rejections.

The information in the above box entails that St John's wort increased the breakdown speed of cyclosporin. This dropped cyclosporin level in the blood, which was confirmed in this man's case.

When the patient was ordered to stop St John's wort by the medical team, his cyclosporin levels were elevated again, and the patient's transplanted liver successfully recovered.

What is counterintuitive about this case is the realization that someone's intent to stay healthy could lead to such a life-threatening event. But many patients self-medicate without talking to their healthcare providers, because they are under the assumption that natural supplements are safe. A survey of 755 transplant patients revealed that more than half of them used nutritional or herbal supplements. A whopping 30% of those who used herbals admitted that they were taking St. John's wort.[44]

Drug interactions with herbs are common. Although these products are not FDA-approved, pharmacists can often recognize important patterns in their interactions (and toxicities).

Let's take a healthy college student, for example, who uses oral contraceptives to prevent pregnancy. Many contraceptives are known to utilize cytochrome P450 enzymes.[45] If she decides to use St John's wort, a similar interaction to the one in the previous case can occur, rendering the birth control pill less effective, and potentially causing her to have an unplanned, unwanted pregnancy.

The purpose of recognizing these issues is not to be deprived of natural remedies that could be used safely. Instead, it is to make an informed decision by talking to a health provider in order to calculate the risks and benefits before starting an herbal supplement. Why go through a life-threatening event when you can predict and prevent it?

Chapter 5
Are familiar and established medications safer than newly approved drugs?

Do you find it easier to trust a drug formulation that has been used for 30 years over a newly released tablet?

Older drugs are less likely to be recalled and cause unexpected outcomes compared to newly approved therapies. The longer a medication is in use, the more data that accumulates to confirm its safety, or to set up monitoring parameters to address any adverse effects. Add to this the comfort factor that comes with familiarity, and it is not surprising that we have a deep-rooted belief that older medications must be safer.

But the assumption that older drugs are safe lead to leniency towards their regulation. Due to this, numerous unapproved drugs bypassed FDA regulations and were used despite never actually being evaluated.

This chapter will shed some light on milestones and shortcomings in drug approval regulations and outline some safety issues associated with older pharmaceuticals.

To further explore these topics, it is best to consider a brief history of drug approval first.

The disturbing incidents of the twentieth century

Drug safety is something we take for granted today. But the FDA's oversight over medications has evolved over the course of many years.

Arguably, the most important period in drug safety started with the erroneously named 'sulfanilamide incident'.

In 1937, more than a hundred people mysteriously died in the United States. They all experienced similar range of symptoms, most of which led to kidney failure. After these cases were thoroughly investigated, a common link was found: an elixir of sulfanilamide.

The strange, deadly effects were entirely unexpected because sulfanilamide is an antibiotic that was frequently prescribed to treat various infections at that time. But the cause of the deaths was not the drug itself. Instead, the poisoning was attributed to a substance used in the elixir formulation.

An elixir is a pharmaceutical preparation that uses a mixture of water and alcohol in carefully controlled proportions. The chemical properties of elixirs make them excellent solvents for some drugs, In the case of sulfanilamide, the elixir contained diethylene glycol (DEG).

Interestingly, elixirs are also used to mask the taste of medications with flavoring. But despite its sweet taste, diethylene glycol was far more sinister than it first appeared.

DEG is a form of alcohol that is metabolized into toxic compounds that cause significant harm to the brain. Exposure can be fatal if not treated urgently. In fact, it is currently used as a component in antifreeze formulations. As you might imagine, its use in drug formulation (e.g., in elixirs) is prohibited now.

The company's pharmacist, Harold Watkin, is said to have committed suicide after he learned about the tragedies caused by his formulation.[46]

At that time, DEG was chosen as a solvent because it helped to dissolve sulfanilamide and tasted sweet. If the pharmaceutical company had carried out proper studies on the toxicities of DEG, the lethality of this ingredient would have been grossly apparent, and preventable. But at that time, it was not required for drugs or ingredients to be reviewed by the FDA for safety before being utilized by patients. This incident had led to the enactment of the Food, Drug, and Cosmetic Act of 1938, which ultimately gave the FDA most of its power to inspect drugs' safety and ensure quality.

Yet another series of disturbing events occurred a few decades later. In the late 1950s, the multi-purpose drug thalidomide was marketed worldwide as safe and effective in the treatment of morning sickness, a common condition that is especially prevalent among pregnant women. But the tragedy of this drug was eventually realized when it resulted in severe birth defects among newborn children. The connection between the incidents and the mothers' exposure to thalidomide was recognized years later. This led to further legislative updates in the United States, namely the Kefauver-Harris Amendment.

Once this act was signed by President Kennedy in 1962, drug safety was forever changed. This act furthered the FDA's scrutiny and mandated that a drug must be proven not only to be safe but also effective before hitting the market. Since that year, companies that wish to develop and market a new drug must have it carefully studied and approved by the FDA for both safety and efficacy.

But with these two major pieces of legislation making great strides in pharmacy practice, we were left with the question of what to do with medications that were already in use.

Grandfathered drugs

When the Kefauver-Harris Amendment was introduced, it was not practical nor economically efficient to evaluate every substance that was already on the market, so medications developed between the 1930s and 1960s had to go through a process called Drug Efficacy Study Implementation (DESI), which required pharmaceutical companies to provide existing information to justify their products' safety and efficacy. In contrast, medications that had been in use before the 1930s were simply 'grandfathered' into the new era based on the assumption that, having been in use for so long, they were safe.

But grandfathered drugs raised a major discrepancy in drug approval process. On one hand, new medications must go through strict evaluation for years, and continue to be studied even after being approved for post-marketing data. On the other hand, grandfathered drugs were able to escape the FDA's formal approval for decades.

Additionally, the use of unapproved drugs raised concerns about drug quality and safety. How would you feel, for instance, if you had been hospitalized for a septic shock, a potentially deadly condition marked by extremely low blood pressure, only to be administered a medication that had never been evaluated by the FDA?

Septic shock is a life-threatening consequence of infections. It is essentially a steep drop in blood pressure. When that occurs, important organs may cease to function as they fail to receive enough blood supply.

Vasopressin is also known as antidiuretic hormone (ADH) because it acts to preserve and reabsorb the fluids that are otherwise lost from the kidney, thereby accumulating fluids, and increasing blood pressure.

As a grandfathered drug, vasopressin was not approved by the FDA despite being used in hospitals for decades. It wasn't until 2011 that a newly branded version of it was submitted for FDA approval.

In 2006, the federal government shifted its position to resolve such discrepancies with a program called the Unapproved Drug Initiative, which pushed to evaluate and approve medications that weren't evaluated before.

But the evaluation process can be very costly (there is more on drug approval process in the next chapter). Given the expense, why would the pharmaceutical industry ever agree to have their products that are already in use put to the test?

In the Unapproved Drug Initiative Guidance of 2011, the FDA declared, "The first company to obtain an approval [of a previously unapproved drug] will have

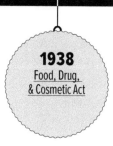

1938
Food, Drug,
& Cosmetic Act

1962
Kefauver-Harris
Amendment

a period of de facto market exclusivity before other products obtain approval."[47] Thus, once a product received approval, all other manufacturers of this product were required to have their (unapproved version of the) product withdrawn from the market.

This system inevitably removed competition for products that got approved. This served as a reward system for manufacturers to voluntarily have their products evaluated.

But without competitive pressure to drive sales, it was consumers who paid the price—in the literal sense.

The cost of the newly approved vasopressin, which used to be cheap, has dramatically increased to about $2,000 per 10ml.[48]

Inflated prices led to shortages of the newly approved vasopressin. Other vasopressin products were removed. Healthcare facilities were not able to maintain a consistent supply of the drug, which was in high demand for COVID-19 patients early in the pandemic.

Now, in contrast to the previous hypothetical scenario, suppose you were hospitalized with septic shock during a more recent time. With the newly approved version of vasopressin, this scenario could play out differently. You may not be able to have access to it or afford it in the first place.

This is how a well-intended program eventually led to unforeseen consequences. In fact, the Department of Health and Human Services (HHS) recently provided a notice of termination of the Unapproved Drug Initiative due to the unexpected shortages. The FDA has not yet formally addressed this issue or initiated a policy in lieu of the initiative.[49]

From a broader perspective, whether we must boost the affordability or availability of urgent therapies at the

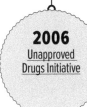

2006
Unapproved
Drugs Initiative

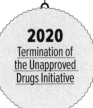

2020
Termination of
the Unapproved
Drugs Initiative

expense of quality is a bioethical dilemma of the current time. It has reached the courts and it continues to divide medical opinions today. At the end of the day, cost matters, but there is also a definite need for quality.

Next is another example of an old drug that raises safety concerns.

Hydroxychloroquine: The curative curse of the cinchona tree

Anyone who paid attention to the news during the COVID-19 pandemic is familiar with the hydroxychloroquine controversy.

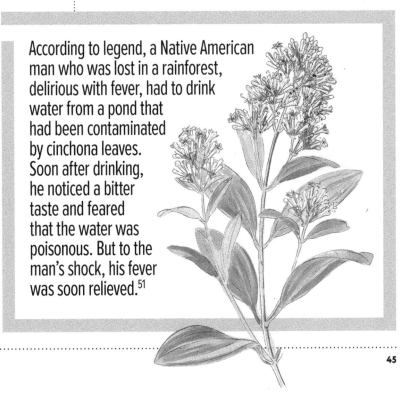

According to legend, a Native American man who was lost in a rainforest, delirious with fever, had to drink water from a pond that had been contaminated by cinchona leaves. Soon after drinking, he noticed a bitter taste and feared that the water was poisonous. But to the man's shock, his fever was soon relieved.[51]

Hydroxychloroquine is traditionally used to treat malaria and autoimmune conditions like lupus. It is now considered a drug that has many untapped potentials.

But what makes hydroxychloroquine particularly interesting is its roots which date back hundreds of years.

The drug is structurally related to quinine, which come from the bark of the cinchona tree. Quinine was used to treat fevers and various conditions as early as the 1600s. It was once called 'Jesuits bark' for its healing powers.[50]

Derivatives of quinine maintained a special popularity across cultures as the go-to cure for malaria. For years, these substances have been edited and synthesized, giving rise to hydroxychloroquine, a synthetic derivative of quinine.

But despite the comforting familiarity we now have about the drug's ancient roots, hydroxychloroquine is not free from risks. Throughout the years, numerous problems have been reported to FDA's adverse drug events monitoring program, Medwatch. Some of the heavily monitored adverse effects include dysregulated heart's rhythm and vision problems (potentially even blindness).[52]

You may report adverse drug events directly to the FDA's Medwatch program using their webpage:[53] www.fda.gov/medwatch/report.htm

---

Chapter 6
Are expensive products better?

People are often presented with a choice between a brand and a generic product.

The sensible decision—at least for most people—is to get the cheaper one. However, sometimes they are left wondering whether the more expensive products offer any advantages that they are neglecting to consider during these transactions.

After all, it is not uncommon to encounter someone who swears by a particular brand product that he or she is willing to pay much higher prices for.

Are these expensive brand products better?

To address this question, this chapter will explore the drug development and approval process in the United States from industrial and legislative standpoints.

A brand-new product

Everyone likes a brand-new something.

In the world of economics, prices are determined by the principle of supply and demand. They fluctuate dynamically to meet the current curve. For instance, if the demand drops for a certain product, its price eventually goes down too.

But unlike most products, prescription drugs must be approved by the FDA before their use. Manufacturers must carry out a rigorous testing process that is both costly and time-consuming. A drug must go through various stages of testing, from the initial development and in-vitro testing, to testing on non-human subjects (often mice), and all the way to clinical trials. This is a process that can take more than a decade, and cost as much as $2.7 billion.[54,55,56] If every company had to go through that process and assume such costs for every product on the market, then we would not have access to many essential medications at affordable prices.

For that reason, the FDA must ensure the availability of affordable medications without sacrificing quality. This is where a generic medication, a cheaper copy of the branded product, comes into play.

Reinventing wheels

Why are brand products more expensive?

Consider the following scenario: company A wants to develop a new medication for arthritis. It submits a new drug application (NDA). After a company spends many years to develop the drug, it spends more years to test it for safety and efficacy. Finally, the company must prove that the drug is safe and efficacious in treating arthritis for thousands of patients in clinical trials. If they can prove that, then company A may receive FDA approval for the drug. Further monitoring will be needed to ensure safety even after approval. Given the exceptional costs, it makes sense that the price set by company A would be high.

After some time, company B may be able to replicate the product. It must show that its product has the same active ingredient, strength, dosage form, and route of administration as the brand drug. But because it requires less investment in developing the drug from scratch, it submits an abbreviated new drug application (ANDA). If granted approval, company B can set a much more affordable price for the drug because it has incurred lower costs. This process balances innovation with competition and allows us to have cheaper options for what is essentially the same drug.

Generic medications can benefit the entire healthcare system by reducing financial burdens for consumers and third-party payers. Like most individuals, insurance companies see little reason to pay higher prices for a medication that offers no unique clinical advantage compared to a cheaper treatment. But insurance companies are at least partially run in collaboration with pharmaceutical scientists or pharmacists themselves, who look for evidence (e.g., trials) before committing to spend on a new medication or make formulary changes. In other words, coming up with a brand-new drug is not only a costly process but also a high-risk endeavor. As a manufacturer, you may get a new drug approved by the FDA, but there is still a chance that

A formulary is a list of medications that are covered by an insurance company.

the drug will not be embraced by third-party payers or preferred in formularies for years.

This is the main reason why using generic medications is a cost-effective strategy. It's a situation in which practically everyone benefits. In fact, about $313 billion was saved in 2019 due to the use of generic medications.[57]

This chapter is primarily focused on budgeting, prices and drug quality. But patients may prefer to take something for reasons other than its price. The complexity of patient preferences goes beyond monetary value. That will be explored more thoroughly in the next chapter.

Chapter 7
Are side effects real or imagined?

Have you ever been told that the side effects you've experienced are not true drug reactions?

Experiencing a side effect that isn't understood or acknowledged can cast doubts in anyone's mind. Odd side effects, like those demonstrated in chapter 1, do indeed occur. Yet, many experts question the legitimacy of reported side effects. This chapter will evaluate whether reactions to drugs are legitimate or simply psychological.

The second part of the chapter will extend that question to consumer preferences in products' appearances or even in choice of manufacturers.

The power of placebo

Doctors have long figured out that anticipation has a special role in medicine. In the 1700s, William Cullen, a physician and influential pharmacologist, used that term when treating a condition that was not curable or when he wasn't confident in his ability to treat a patient.[58] Placebo is Latin for "to please". While the definition of placebo has evolved since then, it still carries a similar connotation in medicine today.[67]

Although placebo is used to collectively describe any anticipated consequence from treatment, the term placebo specifically refers to the expectation of therapeutic effects, whereas nocebo refers to the anticipation of harmful ones.

Nowadays, the placebo effect is utilized in pharmaceutical research, particularly in randomized controlled trials (RCTs). During RCTs, a random portion of participants usually receive an inactive substance in place of the drug. This is usually implemented to distinguish the effect of the active drug from the effect induced by the act of taking a pill (placebo).

Expectations can impact whether a treatment is beneficial or harmful. The question is: to what extent?

It is interesting to apply this question to a controversial subject like the whispered intolerance to the cholesterol lowering drugs, statins.

> Statins lower cholesterol and prevent its buildup in arteries. Specifically, they inhibit an enzyme that produces cholesterol, named HMG-CoA reductase.

By lowering cholesterol, statins have proven to be effective in reducing cardiovascular events like heart attacks.[59]

However, people who are taking statins are commonly observed to experience side effects, particularly muscle pain, stiffness, and fatigue. Many patients, even those facing significant risks of heart attacks or strokes, opt out of statin therapy when they experience severe muscle pain.

But results from RCTs tell a different story. Firstly, side effects appeared much less frequently in studies than those reported in registries or seen routinely in practice. Evidence from these studies certainly does not reflect the prevalence of side effects seen in real life. Secondly, side effects were reported to a similar extent by participants regardless of whether they were receiving statins or placebo.

In other words, participants who took placebo also reported side effects induced by statins like muscle pain.[60,61,62]

Does this mean that the high prevalence of statin intolerance is overestimated? Some health practitioners suspect that muscle pain occurs because patients are conditioned to think about it when they're counseled about statin side effects. But the opinions of experts on statin intolerance are highly polarized. The American College of Cardiology (ACC) published a paper titled "Statin Intolerance: Not a Myth" advising clinicians not to be dismissive of statin complaints and to use a careful approach in evaluating those side effects.[63]

However, as of 2022, the latest and possibly the largest meta-analysis to date, published in the European Heart Journal, found that less than 10% of statin users suffer from side effects— which isn't a low percentage, but it does not match the prevalence observed in practice. The researchers used validated diagnostic criteria to investigate those side effects in more than 4 million people taking statins worldwide. They concluded statin intolerance to be "over-estimated and over-diagnosed".[64,65]

In practice, I see far too many cases of severe muscle pain in statin users to write them off as nocebo effects. Many clinicians also take the results from clinical trials with a grain of salt. In general, an inherent weakness of trials is that they have limited capacity to account for complex real-world data. For instance, it would be challenging to realistically account for drug interactions or for the experiences of special patient populations like the elderly.

Why would these intricate details matter?

Firstly, because drug interactions influence statin levels. Secondly, because certain populations are more sensitive to statin-induced toxicities. Older people, for instance, tend to be excluded from trials.

Nevertheless, what fuels this continuous debate is more than a simple problem of opposing views. Rather, there is also the challenge of distinguishing real side effects from nocebo effects.

A more pressing question that continues to resurface in the medical community is this: can placebo influence a measurable outcome?

When most people talk about benefits of placebo, they refer to improvement in conditions like fatigue or depression, which are challenging to quantify. This creates a common perception about placebo effects that they are "simply psychological".

But placebo can be perceived in a radically different way.

As counterintuitive as it may seem, it is possible that anticipation (of either a reward or an unpleasant effect) can produce a real change in someone's physiology. But this is difficult to prove, especially with outcomes that are not strictly defined or objectively measured.

And this begs us to distinguish between the intrinsic effect of any given drug and its placebo or nocebo effect.

Addressing the blurry lines

A better way to test the placebo effect is to see whether it can influence something that's more clearly defined than pain.

For instance, can placebo lead to different cholesterol levels when patients use statins?

Most researchers don't focus on placebo or adopt it as a main research interest. But Anup Malani, a law professor at the University of Chicago, was solely interested in this question. He wanted to see whether the anticipation of getting the drug (as opposed to the placebo) can lead to a change in cholesterol level, specifically in low-density lipoprotein (LDL) value.

To explore that, he looked at data from different types of trials.[66] In one type, everyone received a statin, whereas in the other trial type, half of the participants were randomly chosen to receive a statin drug while the other half received placebo. It is important to note that the subjects in the second study design did not know which pill they had taken during the study, but they were informed that they had a 50% chance of receiving a placebo pill.

Malani's analysis showed that participants from the trial which did not employ placebo achieved more drastic reductions in LDL level (roughly 25% more reduction) compared to participants who were randomized to receive the active drug in the other study design.

In other words, those who received the treatment with full certainty of getting the drug achieved better results compared to those who received the active drug but were told that they only had a 50% probability of receiving it.

This suggests that you can achieve better measurable results simply by knowing that you have a higher chance of being treated with a drug (compared to placebo).

We are arriving at potential answers here that are substantially different from what we're used to in placebo studies. Needless to mention, if these conclusions are true, they can have broad implications, as they can uncover yet another dimension of our minds' untapped potentials.

So, to answer the question raised earlier in the chapter, it is possible to experience a positive or negative outcome from a drug simply based on our expectations.

The next question is this: can anticipation also influence someone's peculiar preferences in their pills' physical attributes?

Pill pet peeves

Ever notice a change in your pills' shape or color? That happens even if you pick up the exact same medicine from the same pharmacy. It is said that roughly 30% of patients experience these switches at any given year.[68]

Although the FDA requires all generic medications to contain the same active ingredient as the brand product, manufacturers of generic products are not required to replicate the physical appearance of the brand product.

But such changes in pill appearance are concerning to a minority of patients who have strong preferences for a particular pill. In fact, pharmacists are presented with this scenario frequently. Out of the blue, a patient claims that a certain pill color is better suited for them, even though other pills contain the exact same active drug.

This once again leads to the question: what is the fine line between a real side effect and something that is just imagined?

A pill preference or an avoidance tendency tends to develop after a patient has a reaction or bad experience with a particular pill. Interestingly, these issues are less understood or acknowledged because they might be influenced by an inactive ingredient.

For instance, suppose a patient experienced itching from one tablet and asked to switch to a different-looking tablet. Both tablets contain the same dose of the exact same medicine (active ingredient).

If the itch resolves after the switch, it could indicate that something other than the active ingredient might have caused the itch.

What is in the pill anyway?

Oral medications contain other components besides the active ingredients. The complex composition can be appreciated with a simple, binary breakdown.

1. Active ingredient. Active ingredients are, by definition, components that are intended to cause a therapeutic effect. For example, in the case of sulfanilamide, the therapeutic effect was the antimicrobial property that helps fight strep throat.
2. Inactive ingredients. Inactive ingredients are added to a formulation to stabilize the active ingredients, but do not in themselves cause an intended therapeutic effect

Thankfully, the FDA requires inactive ingredients to be studied and thoroughly reviewed for approval before being used. The pharmaceutical industry has accumulated a list of inactive ingredients that have already been reviewed and approved by the FDA and are available to manufacturers to use while developing a medication. For that reason, the existence of inactive ingredients that are entirely novel or unfamiliar is somewhat uncommon, which gives us fewer issues to worry about.

However, just because an inactive ingredient is not therapeutically active does not mean it has zero biological activity.

As a matter of fact, recent reports have linked inactive ingredients to multiple allergic reactions.[69]

Now, returning to the case, an obvious explanation for the itch would be an allergy or a reaction to a component of the first tablet.

But it would be challenging to prove that this was indeed the cause of the itch. It is possible, for example, that the patient was exposed to an environmental trigger when he started the first tablet that ceased to exist after the switch. A coincidence seems unlikely but isn't impossible.

Yet, it's hard to rule out other explanations. For instance, the change in the pill's physical appearance might have given the patient a break and a chance to reset his expectation about the next product. Call it reverse nocebo, if you will.

Consequently, the patient in that scenario can avoid the former pill. Or, he might request the alternate pill with the exact description (color or shape) to avoid further issues.

Interestingly, these situations occur commonly. Many people are told by their providers that their medication reactions or allergies are not real even though they feel real (or *are* real).

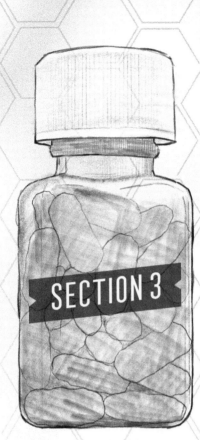

SECTION 3

Pharmacy practice

Chapter 8
Does your pharmacist or physician know your medications?

The healthcare system in the United States currently consists of highly trained, conscientious practitioners.

But it is far from perfect.

This chapter explores common medical mishaps, miscommunications, and errors as well as the current efforts to reduce them.

Consider this case, for instance:

Imagine that you are sent home from the hospital with a new pill, amlodipine (brand name: Norvasc) to treat your high blood pressure. But you start to feel weak and experience personality changes shortly after being discharged.

Your blood pressure begins to spike again. You develop chest pain and eventually get hospitalized for a suspected heart attack. After seeing multiple specialists and undergoing angiography, an invasive procedure to look through your heart's blood vessels, you are only given anxiety and depression pills.

The next few weeks bring further personality changes and intense dizziness. You begin to feel intense light-headedness, and soon you begin having tremors and find yourself unable to stand or walk in an orderly fashion.

Something is off. You don't even feel like yourself anymore.

You are hospitalized for the third time—now for a suspected stroke. Luckily, a CT scan indicates no evidence of stroke. After looking through your medication history, the healthcare team notices that you are taking a medication called Navane.

Navane is the brand name for thiothixene, a first-generation antipsychotic used to treat schizophrenia.

But the issue here is more serious than it looks on the surface.

Dopamine is a neurotransmitter involved in regulating various functions, such as mood, sleep, motivation, movements, and lactation. Thus, preserving "baseline" dopaminergic activity is needed to function properly. For that reason, antipsychotics often come with serious side effects.

First generation antipsychotics are linked to various movement disorders, collectively known as extrapyramidal symptoms (EPS).[70] EPS disorders vary in duration and severity. While some symptoms are reversible, others are chronic and challenging to treat.

The repetitive and involuntary movements that you had experienced in the fictional scenario were the result of this medication blocking your dopamine receptors by binding to the receptors tightly (with high affinity).

The lawsuits filed against manufacturers of Parkinson's disease medicine shed some light on why some people were led to commit impulsive acts.

It would be grossly misleading to over-simplify the pathology behind Parkinson's disease. However, it is worthwhile to consider these intriguing concepts:

Lack of dopamine activity in specific brain regions is often the root of the problem in Parkinson's disease.

As far as dopamine activity is concerned, schizophrenia and Parkinson's disease can be thought to run in opposite directions.

Activating dopamine receptors with dopamine agonists can lead to personality changes and increase in impulsivity. Conversely, blocking dopamine activity by an antipsychotic can lead to movement disorders (possibly mimicking Parkinson's disease).

But how did this medication end up in your possession and why?

After a thorough investigation, it became clear that Navane was initiated in error. You did not have a diagnosis for any condition that would be treated with this medicine. You were simply meant to have received a similarly named drug, Norvasc, to treat high blood pressure. Which points to another realization: throughout the entire time, you never took the medicine you were meant to receive to treat blood pressure.

Now it makes sense. The out-of-control blood pressure, the chest pains, the personality changes, and the movement dysfunction—everything can be traced back to a small innocent mistake that was not caught early enough. This scenario is loosely based on the real-life story of a 71-year-old woman who endured such prolonged turmoil.[71]

In one study conducted at the University of Colorado Hospital, 50 patients were asked to fill out lists of medications they thought they had received during hospitalization. This list was compared to the actual medications they had received. An astonishing 96% of respondents had omitted at least one medication that had been given to them during their stay. Respondents omitted 6.8 drugs on average. 44% truly believed they had received a medication that they had not been given during their stay.[72]

The study has a relatively small sample size. Nevertheless, it can give us an idea of how common this issue is.

Anyone can feel a false sense of security when transitioning from one care setting to another (e.g., being admitted or discharged from hospitals). Patients may not feel the need to ask questions about their medication and may refuse counseling and educational opportunities. As the study shows, a significant portion of hospitalized patients believed that a chronic medication that they took at home, in other words a medication that is likely essential for their health, was being administered to them during their hospital stay, when in fact, it was not.

Medication errors also tend to occur when patients see multiple specialists. People often underestimate the risk of these situations since they feel assured to be receiving care from multiple facilities or medical practitioners. But in fact, it is common for one doctor not to be fully aware of medications given to the same patient by another doctor, potentially leading to deadly errors.

Suboptimal consequences aren't only caused by overt errors. Sometimes, it's the ambiguous directions or papers filled with medical jargon that are given to patients that lead to problems.

A misunderstanding can arise from something as simple as following instructions on a prescription label. Say a woman is being treated for high cholesterol with atorvastatin. A blood test shows alarmingly high levels of low-density lipoprotein (LDL). LDL is known as the "bad cholesterol" for its association with cardiovascular diseases. In response to the test finding, the medical team discusses whether to add a new cholesterol medication to her regimen.

Adding a new drug might sound like a reasonable clinical intervention, but it may lead her to take extra pills unnecessarily, increasing the risk of side effects and further fueling polypharmacy.

What if she, for instance, reveals that she habitually forgets to take atorvastatin?

People forget to take their medicine for various reasons. It is possible, for example, that she gets fatigued and forgetful towards the end of the day, and consequently forgets to take the medicine at bedtime.

Why would she need to take the pill at bedtime in the first place?

Statins were thoroughly discussed in the previous chapter. But a few details were left out.

The enzyme that statins act to inhibit, which synthesizes cholesterol, is generally more active during sleep.

For this reason, the idea that statins must be taken before bedtime has become the standard advice. Most people who take statins are instructed to do so according to the prescriptions labels that they receive.

However, there is another detail about statins that might be exceptionally helpful for this patient.

Atorvastatin is one of the longer-acting statins.[73]

In other words, the woman in this case can take atorvastatin at any time without having to worry about it becoming ineffective later during the day or at night. This would be convenient for her, and it could also help her adhere to a routine which will eventually correct her heightened cholesterol levels.

The irony in this case is that her attempt to strictly follow the label's instructions, without talking to a pharmacist, prevented her from taking the medicine in the first place.

Of course, it is not advisable for patients to ignore instructions; they exist for a reason. Most instructions generated by automated systems suggest taking statins 'at bedtime'. And I haven't yet met a clinician who would question that advice. It is safe to assume that most pharmacists see no reason to diverge from giving generic instructions for statins. It is not inherently wrong, nor harmful, for patients to take a statin medicine at night, after all. But in a case like this, given the medicine's half-life, the woman's high cholesterol level combined with her forgetfulness, a more individualized approach could be taken. This issue could be easily explored if she is presented with a real opportunity to be involved in her healthcare decisions.

"Treat the patient, not the X-ray."

— James M. Hunter [74]

"To err is human"

According to an eight-year study conducted in Johns Hopkins University, around 250,000 patients in the United States die each year due to medical errors.[75]

Such an inordinate statistic is not to be taken lightly. However, it is not realistic to expect health professionals to always refrain from doing something so intrinsic to human nature: making mistakes.

A report released by the Institute of Medicine (IOM) in 1999, titled "To Err is Human: Building a Safer Health System" was a remarkable initiative to change the perceptions that had surrounded medical errors for so long.[76] Rather than blaming individuals for mistakes, which would only discourage them from reporting errors and learning, a much more realistic and practical risk mitigation method must be used.

The Swiss cheese model

The solution is a new way of doing risk assessment. The Swiss cheese model was originally described by James T. Reason and Dante Orlandella at University of Manchester

Imagine passing a marble through slices of Swiss cheese. It may pass a layer or two, but what happens next? Per the Swiss cheese metaphor, a 'mistake' can go undetected by a multi-layered process to the same extent that a marble can pass through layers of Swiss cheese.

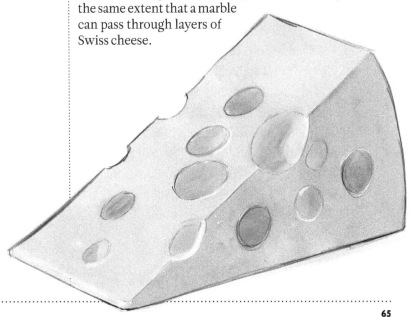

This approach helped shift the blame from individuals because it recognized that health systems can be fragile when it comes to mistakes. It also set realistic expectations to build systems that reduce errors by increasing these 'checkpoints'. The more defense layers (or checkpoints) a system has, the higher the chance that mistakes will be caught, preventing harm to patients.

Examples of those layered 'checkpoints' include asking patients about their medication history, hospitals using software programs that automatically screen for errors, pharmacists monitoring adverse drug events and drug interactions—all the way to the opportunity patients are presented with to speak with their pharmacist at the point of drug dispensation. These are all critical steps that have been put into place to catch errors and prevent harm.

Patients also have a role in preventing errors from happening or from developing into bigger, more harmful issues. Most people can now conveniently communicate questions or concerns with their providers by using technology. Another helpful tactic is to use medication lists.

A medication list has great capacity to prevent medication discrepancies. And it is simple to create—all it takes is to write down all the medications taken regularly, as well as vitamins and supplements.

It is critical that patients share a medication list with pharmacists to screen for continuity and potential interactions. Sharing the list is especially useful during transitions of care.

Another time in which carrying a medication list is crucial is receiving medical care during a critical condition or while being unconscious.

So you have now finished your dive into some of the most interesting and counter intuitive topics in medicine.

And there are surely many more hidden twists and turns still waiting to be discovered.

If any of this has piqued your curiosity, you now know that much of the story is not difficult to uncover. You just need to start with a question.

So where do you want to take it from here?

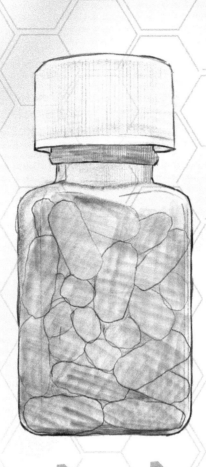

Endnotes

1 Cohen S. M. (1986). Saccharin: past, present, and future. Journal of the American Dietetic Association, 86(7), 929-931.

2 Vane JR (1984). Finding the Right Road. Commencement Address. Valhalla, NY: New York Medical College.

3 Pfizer offers settlement in class action over Parkinson's drug Cabaser. (2014). The Pharmaceutical Journal. Available from: https://pharmaceutical-journal.com/article/news/pfizer-offers-settlement-in-class-action-over-parkinsons-drug-cabaser

4 Mischkowski, D., Crocker, J., & Way, B. M. (2019). A Social Analgesic? Acetaminophen (Paracetamol) Reduces Positive Empathy. Frontiers in psychology, 10, 538. https://doi.org/10.3389/fpsyg.2019.00538

5 Keaveney, A., Peters, E., & Way, B. (2020). Effects of acetaminophen on risk taking. Social cognitive and affective neuroscience, 15(7), 725-732. https://doi.org/10.1093/scan/nsaa108

6 Gervain, J., Vines, B. W., Chen, L. M., Seo, R. J., Hensch, T. K., Werker, J. F., & Young, A. H. (2013). Valproate reopens critical-period learning of absolute pitch. Frontiers in systems neuroscience, 7, 102. https://doi.org/10.3389/fnsys.2013.00102

7 Takeuchi, A. H., & Hulse, S. H. (1993). Absolute pitch. Psychological Bulletin, 113(2), 345-361. https://doi.org/10.1037/0033-2909.113.2.345

8 Levitin, D. J., & Zatorre, R. J. (2003). On the nature of early music training and absolute pitch: a reply to brown, sachs, cammuso, and folstein. Music Percept. 21, 105-110. https://doi.org/10.1525/mp.2003.21.1.105

9 Koren, G., Cairns, J., Chitayat, D., Gaedigk, A., & Leeder, S. J. (2006). Pharmacogenetics of morphine poisoning in a breastfed neonate of a codeine-prescribed mother. Lancet (London, England), 368(9536), 704. https://doi.org/10.1016/S0140-6736(06)69255-6

10 U. S. Food and Drug Administration. Center for Drug Evaluation and Research. (2017). FDA Drug Safety Communication: FDA restricts use of prescription codeine pain and cough medicines and tramadol pain medicines in children; recommends against use in breastfeeding women.

11 U. S. Food and Drug Administration. Center for Drug Evaluation and Research. (2019). Postmarket Drug Safety Information for Patients and Providers: Use of Codeine and Tramadol Products in Breastfeeding Women - Questions and Answers.

12 U. S. Food and Drug Administration. Center for Drug Evaluation and Research. (2017). FDA Drug Safety Communication: FDA restricts use of prescription codeine pain and cough medicines and tramadol pain medicines in children; recommends against use in breastfeeding women.

13 Purdue Pharma. (Revised 2020). Codeine Contin (codeine): Product monograph. Pickering, Ontario, Canada.

14 Dean L, Kane M. (2012). Codeine Therapy and CYP2D6 Genotype. National Center for Biotechnology Information.

15 Chial, H. (2008). DNA Sequencing Technologies Key to the Human Genome Project. Nature Education, 1(1):219.

16 Kaiser, J. (2018). We will find you: DNA search used to nab Golden State Killer can home in on about 60% of white Americans. Science.

17 Spector, N. (2021). Envisioning the FTC as a Facilitator of Blockchain Technology Adoption in the Direct-to-Consumer Genetic Testing Industry, 23 Vanderbilt Journal of Entertainment and Technology Law 679 Available at: https://scholarship.law.vanderbilt.edu/jetlaw/vol23/iss3/6

18 Kumari Chandra V. State of Rajasthan. (2018) (3) RLW 2382 (Raj.)

19 People v. Garcia (2005) 113 P.3d 775 (CO Supreme Court)

20 Qato, D. M., Wilder, J., Schumm, L. P., Gillet, V., Alexander, G. C. (2016). Changes in Prescription and Over-the-Counter Medication and Dietary Supplement Use Among Older Adults in the United States, 2005 vs 2011. JAMA internal medicine, 176(4), 473-482. https://doi.org/10.1001/jamainternmed.2015.8581

21 Sonawane, K. B., Cheng, N., & Hansen, R. A. (2018). Serious Adverse Drug Events Reported to the FDA: Analysis of the FDA Adverse Event Reporting System 2006-2014 Database. Journal of managed care & specialty pharmacy, 24(7), 682-690. https://doi.org/10.18553/jmcp.2018.24.7.682

22 Beers, M. H., Storrie, M., & Lee, G. (1990). Potential adverse drug interactions in the emergency room. An issue in the quality of care. Annals of internal medicine, 112(1), 61-64. https://doi.org/10.7326/0003-4819-112-1-61

23 Bailey, D. G., Spence, J. D., Edgar, B., Bayliff, C. D., & Arnold, J. M. (1989). Ethanol enhances the hemodynamic effects of felodipine. Clinical and investigative medicine. Medecine clinique et experimentale, 12(6), 357-362.

24 Cacabelos R., (2012) World Guide for Drug Use and Pharmacogenomics. EuroEspes Publishing Co. Corunna, Spain.

25 Arbor Pharmaceuticals, Inc. (Revised 2012). E.E.S. ® (ERYTHROMYCIN ETHYLSUCCINATE): PRECAUTIONS - Drug Interactions. Atlanta, GA, USA.

26 MERCK SHARP & DOHME LTD. (2012). ZOCOR (simvastatin) Tablets: DRUG INTERACTIONS. Cramlington, Northumberland, UK.

27 Fallah, A., Deep, M., Smallwood, D., & Hughes, P. (2013). Life-threatening rhabdomyolysis following the interaction of two commonly prescribed medications: a case study. The Australasian medical journal, 6(3), 112-114. https://doi.org/10.4066/AMJ.2013.1616

28 AstraZeneca Pharmaceuticals. (Revised 2014). NOLVADEX (Tamoxifen Citrate): MEDICATION GUIDE. Wilmington, DE, USA.

29 DSM Pharmaceuticals, Inc. WELLBUTRIN® (bupropion hydrochloride): MEDICATION GUIDE. Greenville, NC, USA.

30 BAYER, INC. (Revised 2017). ASPIRIN® 81mg acetylsalicylic acid delayed release tablets USP, 81mg. PRODUCT MONOGRAPH. Ottawa, ON, Canada.

31 Aimo, A., & De Caterina, R. (2020). Aspirin for primary prevention of cardiovascular disease: Advice for a decisional strategy based on risk stratification. Anatolian journal of cardiology, 23(2), 70-78. https://doi.org/10.14744/AnatolJCardiol.2019.89916

32 U. S. Food and Drug Administration. Center for Drug Evaluation and Research. (2011). FDA Drug Safety Communication: Possible increased risk of fractures of the hip, wrist, and spine with the use of proton pump inhibitors.

33 U. S. Food and Drug Administration. Center for Drug Evaluation and Research. (2011). FDA Drug Safety Communication: Low magnesium levels can be associated with long-term use of Proton Pump Inhibitor drugs (PPIs).

34 Hutchinson, W. (1914). The Dawn of the New Doctor. Civilization and Health.

35 Friedlander, Walter J (1992). The Golden Wand of Medicine: A History of the Caduceus Symbol in Medicine. Greenwood Press. ISBN 0-313-28023-1. OCLC 24246627

36 Ondetti, M. A., Rubin, B., & Cushman, D. W. (1977). Design of specific inhibitors of angiotensin-converting enzyme: new class of orally active antihypertensive agents. Science (New York, N.Y.), 196(4288), 441-444. https://doi.org/10.1126/science.191908

37 Eng, J., Kleinman, W. A., Singh, L., Singh, G., & Raufman, J. P. (1992). Isolation and characterization of exendin-4, an exendin-3 analogue, from Heloderma suspectum venom. Further evidence for an exendin receptor on dispersed acini from guinea pig pancreas. The Journal of biological chemistry, 267(11), 7402-7405.

38 Novo Nordisk A/S (2021). WEGOVY (semaglutide): INDICATIONS AND USAGE. Bagsvaerd, Denmark

39 Grieve, M. (1931). A modern herbal; the medicinal, culinary, cosmetic and economic properties, cultivation and folk-lore of herbs, grasses, fungi, shrubs, & trees with all their modern scientific uses. New York :Harcourt, Brace & company.

40 Linde, K., Ramirez, G., Mulrow, C. D., Pauls, A., Weidenhammer, W., & Melchart, D. (1996). St John's wort for depression--an overview and meta-analysis of randomised clinical trials. BMJ (Clinical research ed.), 313(7052), 253-258. https://doi.org/10.1136/bmj.313.7052.253

41 Karliova, M., Treichel, U., Malagò, M., Frilling, A., Gerken, G., & Broelsch, C. E. (2000). Interaction of Hypericum perforatum (St. John's wort) with cyclosporin A metabolism in a patient after liver transplantation. Journal of hepatology, 33(5), 853–855. https://doi.org/10.1016/s0168-8278(00)80321-9

42 Novartis Pharmaceuticals Corp. (Revised 2009). Neoral® Soft Gelatin Capsules (cyclosporine capsules, USP): PRECAUTIONS, Drug Interactions. East Hanover, NJ, USA.

43 Borrelli, F., & Izzo, A. A. (2009). Herb-drug interactions with St John's wort (Hypericum perforatum): an update on clinical observations. The AAPS journal, 11(4), 710–727. https://doi.org/10.1208/s12248-009-9146-8

44 Kaye, A. D., Clarke, R. C., Sabar, R., Vig, S., Dhawan, K. P., Hofbauer, R., & Kaye, A. M. (2000). Herbal medicines: current trends in anesthesiology practice--a hospital survey. Journal of clinical anesthesia, 12(6), 468–471. https://doi.org/10.1016/s0952-8180(00)00195-1

45 Zhang, N., Shon, J., Kim, M.-J., Yu, C., Zhang, L., Huang, S.-M., Lee, L., Tran, D. and Li, L. (2018), Role of CYP3A in Oral Contraceptives Clearance. Clinical And Translational Science, 11: 251-260. https://doi.org/10.1111/cts.12499

46 Kiefer, D. M. (2001). Miracle Medicines: The advent of sulfa drugs in the mid-1930s gave physicians a powerful weapon. TODAYS CHEMIST AT WORK, 10(6), 59-61.

47 U.S. Food and Drug Administration. (2011). Marketed Unapproved Drugs: Compliance Policy Guide Section 440.100. 76 FR 58,398.

48 Regulatory Affairs Professionals Society. (2019). FDA Wins Court Case to Not Put Vasopressin on Compounding List. RAPS website. Available from: https://www.raps.org/news-and-articles/news-articles/2019/8/fda-wins-court-case-to-not-put-vasopressin-on-comp

49 Food and Drug Administration (FDA), Department of Health and Human Services. (2021). Termination of the Food and Drug Administration's Unapproved Drugs Initiative; Request for Information Regarding Drugs Potentially Generally Recognized as Safe and Effective; Withdrawal." Federal Register. Available from: www.federalregister.gov/docu-

ments/2021/05/27/2021-11257/
termina-
tion-of-the-food-and-drug-ad-
ministrations-unap-
proved-drugs-initiative-re-
quest-for-information.
50 Jacoby, D. B. (2005).
Encyclopedia of Family Health,
3rd ed. Marshall Cavendish.
51 Achan, J., Talisuna, A. O.,
Erhart, A. et al. (2011). Quinine,
an old anti-malarial drug in
a modern world: role in the
treatment of malaria. Malaria
journal, 10, 144. https://doi.
org/10.1186/1475-2875-10-144
52 Cadila Healthcare Ltd (Revised
2017). Hydroxychloroquine
Sulfate Tablets, USP: ADVERSE
REACTIONS. India.
53 US Food and Drug
Administration, Center for
Drug Evaluation and Research.
MedWatch: The FDA Safety
Information and Adverse Event
Reporting Program. Available
from: https://www.fda.gov/
safety/medwatch-fda-safety-
information-and-adverse-
event-reporting-program
54 U.S. Food and Drug
Administration. FDA's drug
review process: continued.
Drug review steps simplified.
Available from: http://
www.fda.gov/Drugs/
ResourcesForYou/Consumers/
ucm289601.htm

55 DiMasi, J. A., Grabowski,
H. G., & Hansen, R. W.
(2016). Innovation in the
pharmaceutical industry: New
estimates of R&D costs. Journal
of health economics, 47, 20-
33. https://doi.org/10.1016/j.
jhealeco.2016.01.012
56 Wong, C. H., Siah, K. W., &
Lo, A. W. (2019). Estimation
of clinical trial success rates
and related parameters.
Biostatistics (Oxford,
England), 20(2), 273-286.
https://doi.org/10.1093/
biostatistics/kxx069
57 Association for Accessible
Medicines. (2020). Securing
Our Access and Savings: 2020
Generic Drug & Biosimilars
Access & Savings in the U.S.
AAM Report. Available at
https:// accessiblemeds.org/
sites/default/files/2020-09/
AAM-2020-Generics-
Biosimilars-Access-Savings-
Report-US-Web.pdf
58 Kerr, C. E., Milne, I., &
Kaptchuk, T. J. (2008). William
Cullen and a missing mind-
body link in the early history of
placebos. Journal of the Royal
Society of Medicine, 101(2),
89-92. https://doi.
org/10.1258/jrsm.2007.071005

59 Chou, R., Dana, T., Blazina, I., Daeges, M., & Jeanne, T. L. (2016). Statins for Prevention of Cardiovascular Disease in Adults: Evidence Report and Systematic Review for the US Preventive Services Task Force. JAMA, 316(19), 2008–2024. https://doi.org/10.1001/jama.2015.15629

60 Ridker, P. M., Danielson, E., Fonseca, F. A., Genest, J., Gotto, A. M., Jr, Kastelein, J. J., Koenig, W., Libby, P., Lorenzatti, A. J., MacFadyen, J. G., Nordestgaard, B. G., Shepherd, J., Willerson, J. T., Glynn, R. J., & JUPITER Study Group (2008). Rosuvastatin to prevent vascular events in men and women with elevated C-reactive protein. The New England journal of medicine, 359(21), 2195–2207. https://doi.org/10.1056/NEJMoa0807646

61 Ganga, H. V., Slim, H. B., & Thompson, P. D. (2014). A systematic review of statin-induced muscle problems in clinical trials. American heart journal, 168(1), 6–15. https://doi.org/10.1016/j.ahj.2014.03.019

62 Kashani, A., Phillips, C. O., Foody, J. M., Wang, Y., Mangalmurti, S., Ko, D. T., & Krumholz, H. M. (2006). Risks associated with statin therapy: a systematic overview of randomized clinical trials. Circulation, 114(25), 2788–2797. https://doi.org/10.1161/CIRCULATIONAHA.106.624890

63 American College of Cardiology. (2015) Statin Intolerance: Not a Myth. Expert analysis paper from the American College of Cardiology. Available from: https://www.acc.org/latest-in-cardiology/articles/2015/08/11/09/16/statin-intolerance-not-a-myth

64 European Society of Cardiology. (2022). Statin intolerance is 'over-estimated and over-diagnosed': World's largest study shows less than 10% suffer side-effects caused by the drug. ScienceDaily.

65 Bytyçi, I., Penson, P. E., Mikhailidis, D. P., Wong, N. D., Hernandez, A. V., Sahebkar, A., Thompson, P. D., Mazidi, M., Rysz, J., Pella, D., Reiner, Ž., Toth, P. P., & Banach, M. (2022). Prevalence of statin intolerance: a meta-analysis. European heart journal, ehac015. Advance online publication. https://doi.org/10.1093/eurheartj/ehac015

66 Malani, A. (2006). Identifying placebo effects with data from clinical trials. J. Polit. Econ. 114, 236–256 https://doi.org/10.1086/500279.

67 Cousins, N. (1977). The Mysterious Placebo: How Mind Helps Medicine Work. Saturday Review

68 Kesselheim, A. S., Bykov, K., Avorn, J., Tong, A., Doherty, M., & Choudhry, N. K. (2014). Burden of changes in pill appearance for patients receiving generic cardiovascular medications after myocardial infarction: cohort and nested case-control studies. Annals of internal medicine, 161(2), 96–103. https://doi.org/10.7326/M13-2381

69 Brigham and Women's Hospital & Massachusetts Institute of Technology. (2019). Inactive ingredients in pills and capsules may cause allergic, adverse reactions. Science Translational Medicine.

70 Wubeshet, Y. S., Mohammed, O. S. & Desse, T. A. (2019). Prevalence and management practice of first generation antipsychotics induced side effects among schizophrenic patients at Amanuel Mental Specialized Hospital, central Ethiopia: cross-sectional study. BMC psychiatry, 19(1), 32. https://doi.org/10.1186/s12888-018-1999-x

71 da Silva, B. A., & Krishnamurthy, M. (2016). The alarming reality of medication error: a patient case and review of Pennsylvania and National data. Journal of community hospital internal medicine perspectives, 6(4), 31758. https://doi.org/10.3402/jchimp.v6.31758

72 Cumbler, E., Wald, H., & Kutner, J. (2010). Lack of patient knowledge regarding hospital medications. Journal of hospital medicine, 5(2), 83–86. https://doi.org/10.1002/jhm.566

73 Pfizer Ireland Pharmaceuticals. (2009) LIPITOR® (atorvastatin calcium) Tablets for oral administration: DOSAGE AND ADMINISTRATION. Dublin, Ireland.

74 Hunter JM (1964). Address to the American fracture association.

75 Anderson, J. G., & Abrahamson, K. (2017). Your Health Care May Kill You: Medical Errors. Studies in health technology and informatics, 234, 13-17.

76 Committee on Quality of Health Care in America, Institute of Medicine. (2000). To Err is Human: Building a safer health system. National Academy Press, Washington, D.C.

Milton Keynes UK
Ingram Content Group UK Ltd.
UKHW040917041224
3396UKWH00018B/76